THE HYGIENE COOKING: CLEAN EATING

perfect Cookbook for a Healthy fits

BY

CORINE R. HART

Neither in part or in full can the document be copied, scanned, faxed or retained without approval from the publisher or creator.

TABLE OF CONTENTS

Introduction

Eating clean and healthy is one

of the issues that many people

confront in our country and

throughout the world today. A

clean diet is crucial for excellent

health and nutrition, as it protects

you from chronic diseases.
Healthy eating is a long-term
plan to eat healthier.
It is not a severe diet to follow
for a limited period. A healthy
diet requires no special foods.
Instead, it covers items that are
widely available and generally
known to you.
 Healthy eating include eating a
variety of foods every day and
consuming more of the foods that
offer energy and Crucial
resources that our body system
needs for a smart and healthy
life, and less foods that are low
in nutrition.

Most people get ailments because they are unable to eat clean.

If you've recently been diagnosed with a condition, you're undoubtedly wondering, "Okay, now what do I eat or how do I prepare my meals?" Or, if you've had diabetes for a while and have decided to incorporate healthy eating into your management strategy, you might be wondering, "Where do I start?" Worry no more, sweetie, since this book will provide you with a better understanding and ideas for where and how to begin creating those mouthwatering meals you have always desired. Remember, health is wealth.

CHAPTER 1
Clean and Slow

Cooking healthy is a sure monitoring enquiry carried out by WHO shows it is mostly hygienic to prepare large cuts of meat and poultry using a slow cooking method. Follow the manufacturer's recipes and safety guidelines. Start clean. Starting with a more uninfected and sanitized hands, household appliances and also a clean cooker.

When preparing meat;

Thaw first. Be sure you warm meat or poultry before placing them in a clean cooker. If refrigerated pieces are utilized

they must not hit 140^{0}F speedily
enough and could result to
illness.

Preheat the cooker and, if
feasible, pour in hot liquids.
Adequately heating the pot
earlier enough and applying the
contents or cooking using the
highest point for the first three to
four hour will enable a rapid
burn and reduce the duration
items are in the danger zone.
This is especially important
when cooking meat or poultry in
a slow cooker. Do not cook on
warm. Avoid using the slow heat
setting to prepare food. It is
intended to keep cooked food
hot.

When cooking beans;

Soak and boil dry beans first.
Dried beans, particularly
kidneys, contain a natural toxin.
These poisons can be quickly

destroyed by boiling temperatures. Soak beans for 12 hours, drain, and boil on the stovetop for at least 10 minutes before putting them in a slow cooker.

When cooking vegetables

Place vegetables on the bottom or sides. Vegetables cook slowly, so arrange them near the heat, on the bottom and sides of the slow cooker.

Keep the lid on. During the cooking period, do not lift the lid or cover more than is necessary. When the lid is raised, the internal temperature lowers by 10 to 15 degrees, slowing the cooking process by 30 minutes. Check with a food thermometer. Before consuming meat or poultry, use a food thermometer to ensure that it has achieved a safe internal temperature to eliminate microorganisms. Roasts should be cooked between 145°F to 160°F.

Poultry: 165 degrees Fahrenheit.

Soups, stews, and sauces: 165 degrees Fahrenheit.

Allow to cool properly. Do not leave cooked food to cool in the crockpot. Eat immediately or store leftovers.

Avoid reheating in a slow cooker Do not reheat food or leftovers in a slow cooker; instead, reheat on the stove or in the microwave (165 degree F or higher) then transfer to the slow cooker to keep warm (140 degree F or above).

CHAPTER 2: Stocks, Broths, and Sauces

Learning different stocks, sauces, and soups is vital for anyone trying to construct their menu. Before you can create fresh and unusual foods, you must first learn how to make stocks, sauces, and soup. These three provide a foundation for culinary innovation.

An introduction to various stocks, sauces, and soups. Stocks, soups, and sauces form the backbone of numerous cuisines around the world. Award-winning dishes at five-star restaurants begin with any of these three ingredients. Here's a quick overview of these three dish bases:

Stocks are savory liquids that serve as the foundation for soups, sauces, and other foods.

These are often made by cooking beef, fish, or fowl flesh and bones, vegetables, and seasoning in liquid. Using bouillons and stock bases such as Knorr Beef Broth Base or Knorr Chicken Cubes may easily improve your stocks with rich, meaty tastes, reducing cooking time and increasing efficiency.

Types of stocks in cooking

Brown stock is made by cooking beef or veal bones in a lightly greased roasting pan in the oven.

White stock is often made by using stew and unbrowned veau or brisket bones which produce more delicate flavors.

Chicken stock is made by boiling chicken bones with mirepoix and seasonings. It is also known as "white stock."

Fish stock is made from the bones, heads, skins, and trimmings of lean, white deep-sea fish.

Soups should be made with high-quality ingredients and correct processes. The "body" of the soup is made of gelatine from cooked bones, but meat, fish, poultry, or vegetables can also be used as thickeners. There are two types of soups:

1. Clear soups.

Clear soups are basic, containing no solid components. Here are several examples:

The broth is a flavorful liquid produced as a byproduct of cooking meat or vegetables.

Vegetable soup is a liquid made from clear seasoned stock or broth mixed with one or two types of cooked vegetables. Consommé is a rich, savory stock or broth that has been made clear and translucent.

2. Thick soups.

This soup differs from transparent soups in that it is opaque. Thick soups are heavier because they contain thickening ingredients like roux. For a thicker consistency, combine one or more pureed items into the mixture. It creates the following: Cream soup is a liquid that has been thickened with a roux or other thickening agents, usually milk or cream.

Puree - A soup that is naturally thickened by one or more pureed components or is made with starchy elements.

Chowder is a hearty American-style soup made with fish, shellfish, or vegetables.

Potage - A thick and hearty soup or stew made up of meats or vegetables simmered in liquid to achieve a thick consistency.

Sauces

Sauces are liquids that add flavor and palatability to food, as well as improve its appearance, nutritional value, and moisture content.

Most fried, grilled, roasted, and steamed dishes benefit from a variety of sauces. Sauces can be made in a variety of ways, but the following thickeners are particularly effective:

Slack or brown roux - To thicken demi-glace sauces, use more fat than flour.

Lean or white roux: Make with more flour than grease. This can be combined with milk to make béchamel sauce, or with meat stock to make velouté.

Egg - Use a full egg because the whites keep moisture loosely for a creamy texture and the yolk adds thickening strength.

Use starch derived from waxy maize, corn, potato, or rice. Dissolve the starch in hot water to create gelatinization for a suitable thickener.

Sauce Types

Brown sauce is made with mirepoix, lard, and flour to produce a tan-colored sauce.

Veloute sauce is derived by adding white stock with roux to make a base for creamy soups and vegetable sauces.

Béchamel sauce is made with flour, butter, and milk from a meat foundation.

The cream sauce is made using rich cream or a milk base to create a white liquid.
Preparing any of these liquids will take practice because they are not easy to master. Your first try may not even produce the desired results. To save time and effort, try Knorr Chicken Cubes or Knorr Beef Broth Base. These goods taste similar to homemade stocks, sauces, and soups.

CHAPTER 3

Beans and grains

Today we'll look at beans, rice, and other grains, which are the go-to ingredients for competent cooks everywhere. These simple pantry basics are easy to keep on hand and, when prepared properly, are extremely gratifying and healthful. If you've ever wondered if you need to soak those red kidney beans for so long, or if that side of rice on your plate could be a bit more flavorful, now is your day.

Why Grain and Beans?

You probably have a bag or two of rice and some canned beans in your kitchen cupboard right now. There can be seemingly some dried beans and quinoa. And it's possible that whatever way you use to cook these staples, you learned them a long time ago and, aside from double-checking ratios.

It's a shame Beans and grains are more than just dinner accompaniments, soup fillers, or a method to transform a few pieces of sesame chicken into a substantial dish. They are great main dishes in and of themselves, with plenty of flavor and a full base of protein, fiber, and nutritious carbohydrates.

Beans of All Sorts

First and foremost, let's clarify: Canned beans are excellent! They're practical, affordable, simple to use, and taste good. I mean, they are fine. In terms of flavor and variety, however, dried beans just cannot be compared.

There are dozens upon dozens of dried beans, ranging from adzuki to yellow eye, each with its distinct flavor and texture. And, when you cook them yourself, you may flavor them with a variety of aromatics spices. Each has a place. If you need to cook something quickly on a weekday, open a can. However, if you want to make a special dish for a party or simply something a little nicer, it may be worthwhile to soak and cook dry beans.

If you've never made dried beans from scratch, especially an heirloom type, you're in for a quiet mind-blowing culinary discovery. Cooking beans from home produces a saucy "pot liquor" and deep, surprising flavors that can equal meat in terms of enjoyment and depth.

In terms of the beans themselves, you're undoubtedly familiar with the following varieties:

There are medium-sized beans, including **black beans, scarlet beans, chickpeas, and kidney beans.**

Then there are little beans like split peas and other lentils. Finally, there are large beans such as **fava, lima, and Royal Corona beans.**

Bean flavors can vary widely depending on the type—chickpeas are nutty and slightly sweet, green lentils are grassy and earthy, and black beans are umami-rich and earthy. When cooked properly, beans should be beautifully creamy but firm, with no grittiness. If you do not like one flavor, try another—there are plenty to choose from.

Grains of all sorts

Let's start with the fundamentals here. Grain refers to the seeds or kernels of cereal crops such as wheat, rice, barley, and sorghum. (Observe how grain travels from field to bread.) The "whole grain" includes the outer bran, endosperm, and germ, all of which are edible.

White rice and pearled barley are examples of highly milled grains, which have had the outer hull and most of the germ removed. They have less nutritional content, but they cook faster and, according to some, taste better. Whole grains are normally brown, whereas milled grains are white or very light brown.

Why Should You Rinse Dried Beans and Grains?

Most grains and beans available for purchase should be washed before cooking, not just because they are likely dusty from time spent in processing facilities and factories (which they are), but also because it results in a better-tasting dish in the end. Rinsing removes some of the starch from the grain's surface (especially rice), making it less sticky. To rinse rice, simply place the grains in the pot you're using, add water, swirl it around with your hand, drain, and repeat until the water runs clear.

Rinsing can eradicate components which leads quinoa to taste stinky. Typically, your recipe will mention whether or not the grains should be washed. And, nearly typically, canned beans must be rinsed to remove the thick canning liquid before use in a dish.

Why Do Most Recipes Call for Soaked?

While small beans, such as lentils, do not require soaking, medium- and large-sized beans should be soaked in three to four inches of lukewarm water and a pinch of baking soda then left at room temperature for six to eight hours — or overnight — before cooking. Baking soda tenderizes the skins, making them simpler to digest.

Do you need to soak dry beans before cooking them? No. Most beans can be cooked in the oven, Instant Pot, or stovetop pressure cooker without presoaking — or with a shorter fast soak — and will still be edible.

However, there are various benefits to soaking them (and if time is an issue, you may want to use canned).

Soaking dry beans reduces active cooking time significantly. They will also grow to around 2.5 times their original size, making them considerably easier to stomach. (Considering beans' well-deserved reputation for creating flatulence, this is significant).

This results in a far better
ingredient for soups, stews, and
bean salads. (If you're making
chickpeas, you may use the
leftover bean water as a vegan
egg white substitute.
If You Only Learn One Thing
Today...
To get the most flavor out of any
grain you're cooking, toast it
first—from rice and barley to
millet and steel-cut oats.
Toasting dried grains on a sheet
pan in the oven takes about 15
minutes, results in a much richer
flavor, and has the added benefit
of having your entire house smell
great. Simply preheat.
Preheat the oven to 350°F,
arrange them evenly on a baking
sheet, and take them out when
they start to smell toasty and
nutty. Grains can even be toasted

directly in the saucepan; here are instructions for oats.

Believe it or not, you don't need to study or even be concerned about water ratios when cooking grains on the stove. The majority of grains can be cooked just like pasta.

With rice, you can use the spaghetti approach or an equally simple trick: the one-knuckle method. Pour the rice into the pan, level it, and touch the top with your finger.

Then pour water till it reaches your first knuckle. That is sufficient water for the majority of pot sizes. Neat!

Okay! We've covered the basics of selecting and preparing beans and grains for cooking. Now let's talk about how to make them taste good.

First, and perhaps most painfully, aim to make boiling beans a project: The type and size of beans you use, as well as their age, will influence how long they take to tenderize. Beans continue to dry out with age, so "fresher" dried beans cook faster.

When you have a saucepan boiling on the stove, check it now and then by removing a bean and tasting it to determine whether it is done.

Second, flavorings are beneficial to both beans and grains. This begins with adding salt to the liquid before cooking (yes, even the bean water should be salted), but it doesn't have to end there. Grains absorb the liquid they are cooking in, so don't limit yourself to simple water: Broth or stock may provide a lot of depth, as can coconut water or

almost any other liquid, from
fruit juice to tea! Stock doesn't
have much of an impact on bean
flavor, but adding aromatics like
bay leaves, onion, garlic cloves,
or herbs makes a tremendous
difference, and the resulting
liquid virtually becomes a broth
in its own right!
And after they're done frying,
taste them and start adding
additional flavor:
 Consider the flavors in the rest
of your meal.
Make, then look for
complementing additions.
Perhaps a little acid, like lemon
juice or tomato. Perhaps a hint of
sweetness from brown sugar or
maple syrup. Peradventure the
pots need an additional salt, drop
a pinch of it at a time by making
it taste as you desire. Finally, to
prevent beans from overcooking,

splitting, or coming apart, immerse the entire pot in an ice bath in the sink. They will swiftly cool in their liquid, keeping the ideal texture. Extra beans can be refrigerated in their liquid form or frozen in containers for extended storage. Cooked grains can also be frozen easily.

CHAPTER 4: Breakfast and Brunch.

A healthy breakfast not only gives you the energy you need to stay active throughout the day, but it also jumpstarts your metabolism. Furthermore, a healthy and hearty breakfast regulates blood sugar levels, aids in weight management, enhances cognitive function, and promotes heart health. However, eating fruit on the move or drinking a glass of juice does not give adequate nourishment. Here, we'll talk about what makes breakfast nutritious and when is the best time to have breakfast.

Does Breakfast Time Matter?

Eating a nutritious breakfast is not sufficient.

To reap the most benefits, eat a nutritious, hearty breakfast at the appropriate time. When you eat breakfast is just as important as what you eat for breakfast.

Eating breakfast at the appropriate time sets the tone for a balanced appetite and maintains blood sugar levels throughout the day. When you eat late, your blood sugar levels rise, causing hunger and cravings that contribute to overeating.

When we wake up, our bodies need to speed up and break the fast so that we can stay energetic throughout the day.

So, what is the right time to take your breakfast?

The perfect moment to take breakfast is between two to three hours of waking up.

To enhance our metabolism, we should consume breakfast by 8:00 a.m. Waiting till 9 or 10 a.m for breakfast is too late and won't provide the necessary benefits.

Eating breakfast at the appropriate time boosts your mental and physical performance throughout the morning, which is the most productive time of the day. Eating breakfast on time also helps to control your late-night cravings.

What if you exercised in the morning?

Many people go to the gym in the morning before starting their day. Even if you go to the gym in the morning, make sure to eat something light before working out. For example, you can consume oatmeal before you go to the gym. Your body is in healing mode following an exercise session because your muscles are regenerating. This is why you should eat a second breakfast with vegetables or lean proteins.

A light mid-morning snack, such as boiled eggs or a sandwich, will keep you satisfied until noon. KENT Sandwich Toaster allows you to make your favorite stuffed sandwiches in minutes.

What Are the Benefits of Eating Breakfast on Time?

Eating breakfast on time has several health and wellness benefits. Here are some benefits connected with eating breakfast at the right time:

1. Improves Metabolism: Eating breakfast after a fast boosts metabolism, allowing for more efficient calorie burn throughout the day.

2. Energy: Breakfast provides important nutrients and glucose, allowing for a strong start to the day and efficient performance of everyday duties.

3. Improves Cognitive Function: Eating a nutritious breakfast provides glucose to brain cells, leading to improved concentration, memory, and performance.

4. Weight Control: Eating breakfast can lead to better weight management. Breakfast

can help with weight
management because it prevents
overeating later in the day.

**5. Improves Nutrient
Intake:** Breakfast provides an
opportunity to consume vital
nutrients including fiber,
vitamins, minerals, and proteins
that may be deficient in other
meals.

**6. Balances Blood Sugar
Levels:** Eating a balanced
breakfast with complex
carbohydrates, proteins, and
healthy fats will help stabilize
blood sugar levels and prevent
energy dips and cravings.

7. Improves Mood: Eating
breakfast can boost mood and
emotional well-being. Skipping
breakfast can cause low blood
sugar levels, irritability, and
mood swings.

8. Improves Digestion: A well-balanced breakfast can stimulate the digestive system and encourage regular bowel movements, leading to improved gut health.

9. Improves Nutritional Choices: Eating a nutritious breakfast can lead to improved eating habits throughout the day, reducing the likelihood of harmful snacks and dinners.

10. Promotes Heart Health: A balanced breakfast with whole grains, fruits, and nuts can help preserve cardiovascular health.

11. Lowers Risk of Chronic Diseases: Eating a nutritious breakfast regularly has been linked to a lower risk of chronic diseases, including type 2 diabetes and obesity.

12. Encourages Physical Activity: Breakfast offers energy for exercise, making it simpler to stay active.

Last Few Words

Because breakfast is the most essential meal of the day, you must not only eat properly but also at the appropriate time.

 Indulging in a late breakfast is worthless because you will not benefits in the importants of a perfect and healthy breakfast. Eating breakfast at the proper time is essential for keeping healthy, whether it's to kickstart your metabolism or to keep your blood sugar levels stable.

What about brunch?

A traditional brunch consists of several parts, reflecting the fact that it is intended to serve both breakfast and lunch at the same time. As a result, many people identify it with the weekend, particularly Sundays. Perhaps this is because many individuals can sleep on the weekends, so a late breakfast or an early lunch is more appealing to folks at this time of day.

What can you have for brunch?

Eggs: For brunch, you can serve fried eggs, eggs Benedict, omelets, and even breakfast burritos.

Bread is another popular brunch staple, along with French toast, pancakes, waffles, and other bread-based dishes like burgers and sandwiches.

CHAPTER 5
Sides

Side dishes can enhance the meal experience and add variety. So, if you're weary of

eating the same dull meals every

day, a side dish can help. But

what if I tell you that a simple

side dish might not only add

flavor to your meals, but also

provide a boost of vitamins,

minerals, and antioxidants? So,

here are a few simple side dish

options offered by health experts

to enhance your meal game.

**Asparagus with Balsamic
Sauce :**
Asparagus contains vitamin K,
fiber, and folate, making it an
excellent healthy side dish. To
make this dish more delightful,

make a flavorful Balsamic sauce and serve it over baked asparagus.

To improve the flavor and nutritional value of this dish, add some roasted garlic.

Kale with toss:

Tossed vegetables are delicious with any meal, but what distinguishes this delicacy is the nutrient-dense combination of Kale and white beans. This Kale and White Bean salad is high in fiber, iron, folate, and protein and tastes great when tossed with olive oil, garlic, and mild seasonings.

Roasted garlic with mashed potatoes:

This may surprise you, but health experts feel that adding a tiny bit of mashed potatoes to your meals can increase their nutritional value. Potatoes include plenty of vitamin B6 and vitamin C, as well as protein, fiber, and carbs. To make this delectable side dish, combine fat-free cream and roasted garlic.

The addition of fresh low-fat cream reduces saturated fat and makes the dish far healthier than fried or baked potatoes loaded with butter.

Creamy and Nutty Coleslaw: Pair your simple dishes with Creamy & Nutty Coleslaw, made with raw cabbage, shredded carrots, cream, and mild spices. The inclusion of cabbage makes it ideal for digestion, while the addition of carrots makes the food high in antioxidants. According to studies, eating raw cabbage daily may help prevent cancers such as prostate, colon, and breast. Serve this dish with sandwiches, burgers, and beef steaks, and top with a handful of roasted peanuts for extra protein.

Sauteed Green Beans:

Sautéed green beans are a delicious and healthful side dish to serve with any dinner. Fiber is high in nutrients and low in calories. Sauté them with red onions, garlic, ginger, and mild spices before topping with parmesan cheese and serving hot with meals. Enjoy!

Baked sweet potatoes:

This side dish will never disappoint. Baked Sweet Potatoes are high in minerals, fiber, and antioxidants, making them an ideal low-calorie side dish. Simply arrange sweet potatoes on a baking dish and brush with a mixture of olive oil, mixed herbs, pepper, salt, and paprika before baking to perfection. Pair these with any meal and enjoy the goodness.

CHAPTER 6

soups and

stews.

A cup of soup or stew might be the ideal comfort food: it's warm, filling, and full of nutrients. But, do yourself a favor and keep the canned ones for emergencies. Though convenient, they frequently include significant amounts of hidden sugars and other ingredients, which might disturb metabolic health.

First, add flavor using veggies and aromatics. Mirepoix is a mixture of chopped celery, carrots, and onions sautéed in butter and oil that is commonly used as the initial step in soup recipes. Do not neglect this step; it is the foundation of taste in your soup.

Use a good broth. "A perfect soup needs stocks with numerous flavor," As was stated by Alexander. "For some, that can imply peppery. For others, it simply implies a combination of elements. To accomplish this, make a stock from scratch with an abundance of aromatics (such as mirepoix, garlic, or Japanese chilies). If using a store-bought broth, consider a high-quality bone broth produced by patiently simmering grass-fed/pastured bones (such as FOND, Kettle & Fire, or Bonafide).

Incorporate as many low-carb, micronutrient-dense vegetables as possible. Kale, spinach, carrots, and zucchini are all great choices, but you have options. Check out this list for inspiration. Keep in mind that some vegetables go mushy, so don't add them until you're almost ready to serve the soup. Asparagus is a great example. Kale and other hard greens, on the other hand, can withstand longer cooking times.

For even more vegetables, bury them in the soup base. If you or a family member dislikes cooked vegetables, consider incorporating them into your soup. Cauliflower is particularly flexible, but kale and spinach can be hidden when combined into a soup base.

Reduce intake of carbohydrates, which can induce blood glucose spike leading to diabetes. Potatoes, corn, squash, and peas have a higher glycemic index and may cause a glucose surge in some persons. Consume these high-starch items in moderation, and make sure to balance them with fat and protein.

Select high-quality proteins. Beans and legumes provide lean protein and fiber, although they can cause surges in some people. Pairing them with fat, such as olive oil or meat, can help to soften the spike. Look for meats that are organic, grass-fed, and responsibly sourced.

Avoid traditional noodles, rice, and other grains. These are high in carbohydrates and may cause glucose spikes. Instead, consider pasta options that are less likely to cause blood sugar spikes.

Use just enough salt. There is no way around it, broth-based soups require only salt. However, don't go overboard with salt while cooking; season to taste when the soup is almost ready to serve.

Avoid added sugars. Homemade soups do not require extra sugar. Vegetables such as carrots, butternut squash, and tomatoes are naturally sweet.

Experiment with other herbs and spices, such as turmeric, cinnamon, basil, pepper, and others, to add taste while also providing antioxidant protection. The recipes below can help you get started, but feel free to change the spice amounts to your preference.

Take the time to cook properly. If a recipe specifies a simmer, follow the instructions.

Eat after your meal. Some soups, such as tomato or squash, may trigger a large glucose increase in some persons.

A well prepared meal as part of a balanced diet with numerous of goodly lipids and proteins (taken first) can help control intense blood glucose spikes.

CHAPTER 7: Vegetables and more vegetables:

As people become more health-conscious, they tend to choose leafy green vegetables over sauce-heavy meats.

Raw vegetables are excellent. Raw vegetables are an excellent alternative for eaters who enjoy "getting back to nature". Serve these in salads with a light sauce for a delightful snack, or add some meat to turn a nutritious salad into a full meal.

Cooked veggies are also good. There are certain advantages to cooking your vegetables.

Cooking, for example, can enhance the antioxidant content in foods like tomatoes and broccoli.

Cooking can also act as a catalyst, releasing nutrients that would be unavailable if taken raw.

Different methods to prepare your vegetables.

Roasting/baking:

Roasting or baking vegetables is an excellent technique to cook them while maintaining the majority of their nutrients. Since the vegetables are not cooked in water, the nutrients contents do not percolate into water.

Steaming:

Steaming has been hailed as the best way to cook vegetables because it uses very little water. Steaming, like roasting and baking, is a fat-free cooking method since it requires no additional oils or fats. That's a double benefit for health-conscious diners worried about their waistlines and hearts.

Slow cooking:

Vegetables cooked in a slow cooker or crock pot keep more of their natural vitamins and nutrients than harsher cooking methods, such as boiling, due to the lower temperatures. Although prolonged cooking in crock pots allows certain nutrients to escape into the water, most people use them for soups and stews, consuming the nutrient-rich liquid alongside the veggies.

We recommend putting your vegetables in the slow cooker near the conclusion of the cooking time after the meat has been simmering all day. This will help to prevent some unneeded nutrition loss in the slow cooker.

Stir- frying:

Stir-frying (or sautéing) preserves some of the vitamins and nutrients in your vegetables while adding fat.

To keep vegetables as healthy as possible, use healthy fats such as olive oil instead of fat-laden oils.

If keeping nutrients is important, boiling vegetables may not be the best option.

This is because boiling extracts vitamins, minerals, and nutrients from the vegetables and into the cooking water. When the veggies are finished cooking, the water is frequently drained and discarded, essentially flushing all of the beneficial vitamins and nutrients. With the proper knowledge and technique, it is possible to prepare recipes that are both nutritious and delicious.

So cook your vegetables correctly, and your health-conscious customers will be eager to return for more - and they'll probably tell all their friends about your "delicious" menu.

CHAPTER 8

seafood and poultry.

Paella in the slow cooker? Yes! The simple and healthful paella recipe calls for chicken and shellfish and cooks in just a few hours.

Of course, you may prepare paella in the slow cooker. As I've previously stated, I believe practically anything can be produced in the slow cooker. There are so many variations of paella out there: seafood,Chicken, combination, vegetarian, etc. Everyone has their own interpretation and/or perspective on what constitutes a true paella.

The slow cooker seafood is prepared in a flexible kitchen device that allows food to stew for a longer amount of time.

A crockpot also known as a slow-cooker, is typically constructed of a ceramic or porcelain pot that is enclosed in an electric heating element. Slow cooking helps flavors to mingle and develop, making it great for creating delectable and soft foods, including fish and seafood.

Fish and seafood are among the most exciting culinary excursions. A sweet and flaky fish filet is simple to prepare and tasty when done properly.

 Scallops are the simplest form of luxury, and shrimp is our go-to option for a quick and fancy date night. But fish can be pricey and complex, right? If you've ever hesitated at the fish counter, read a recipe for fish tacos, wondered how red snapper differed from tilapia, or simply stared at a dry, miserable dish of salmon and wondered what went wrong, this book is for you!

Here's what to purchase, how to cook it, and other techniques to make fish the most confident, exciting component of your repertoire.

Take a clean bowl, place it in the sink, and fill it with cold water. (To prevent bacteria growth, let the water flow slightly or swap it every five minutes.)

And if you haven't planned anything for supper but have filets in the freezer, you can skip the thawing step and cook them right away. Of course, they will require more cooking time than thawed fish. And the oven is the best source of heat. However, it is possible to obtain results that are just as soft and flaky as they were completely thawed.

There are several techniques you can prepare your fish.

Marinating Fish:

Marinating fish is an excellent technique to cook it if you have the time to plan. This works very

well with salmon, and for many
of the reasons why poaching is
so successful:
The marinade adds moisture and
prevents the fish from drying out.
However, it also allows you to
dry-cook the fish for a somewhat
crispy surface. Miso, sugar, oil,
and other spices make an
excellent marinade for fish.

Broiling fish:

Broiling — cooking food over a
high heat source in the oven — is
an excellent technique to
simulate the effects of grilling or
open-fire cooking indoors.
The food is brought very close to
a hot source of heat, with no pan
or dish in the way. And it is
simple: You turn on the oven's
broiler (on some stoves, broiling
takes place in a separate
compartment under the oven),
and when it's hot enough, you

just put a tray of fish in as close to the heat as possible.

Chicken is a global household staple.

It's a great source of animal protein and is high in B vitamins, iron, potassium, and selenium.

Chicken meat is highly adaptable and can be prepared in a variety of ways. However, not all chicken cooking methods are equivalent in terms of health advantages.

This slow-cooked, low-temperature approach minimizes nutrition loss and yields delicate chicken with high mineral content.

You can utilize specify sous vide equipment, but a clean slow cooker and a water bath are more adequate.

How to prepare sous vide chicken at home.

Add flavor to raw chicken and store it in a clean container, free plastic bag or sous vide sack.

Fill a pot with water and attach a thermometer to the side of it. Alternatively, dip a thermometer into the water as needed to monitor the temperature while cooking.

Bring the water to 140^0F (60^0), then add the wrapped chicken bag to the pot. The temperature may drop when you add the meat, so wait until it reaches 140^0F (60^0C) again before beginning the timer.

Set a timer for one hour once the water temperature has restored to 140^0F (60^0C). You can choose to sear the finished meat or simply cut and serve.

CHAPTER 9
Pork and Beef

Slow cookers are an excellent way to prepare pork shoulder. Even your favorite restaurant cannot compete with that melt-in-your-mouth beef. Whether you're craving luscious slow-cooked pulled pork or something more daring, we've got every slow-cooker pork shoulder recipe you'll ever need, from sticky Asian-style dishes to hot Mexican soups.

The greatest pig chops for slow cookers

There are numerous ways to enjoy pork in your slow cooker, ranging from entire pig joints with plenty of fat and connective tissue to leaner diced pork, pork mince, or loin.

Each cut takes slightly different preparation or cooking times, so continue reading to learn how to manage your preferred pig cut. Pork makes an excellent choice for a low-calorie lunch or dinner recipe. Lean pork tenderloin, chops, and roasts can be included in a healthy diet in the form of a shredded pork sandwich, a roasted pork salad, or a fulfilling pork stir-fry.

How to cook pork chops:

Step 1

Heat 2 teaspoons of oil in a large frying pan over medium-high heat.

Step 2

Add the pork and cook for 3-4 minutes per side for medium, or until done to your preference.

Step 3

Transfer to a plate and wrap with foil. Set aside 5 minutes to rest. Serve with your desired sauce or side dish.

How long does it take to cook pork chops?

A pork chop around 2.5cm thick will take about 6 minutes to cook on medium to high heat. Peradventure the pork chop weighs above 2.5cm, it will turn pink when prepared or put in the slow cooker. If you want the chop to be white on the interior, simply increase the cooking time on each side by about a minute. Slow cookers are an excellent way to prepare pork shoulder. Even your favorite restaurant cannot compete with that melt-in-your-mouth beef.

Whether you're in the mood for luscious slow-cooked pulled pork or something more daring.

There are numerous ways to enjoy pork in your slow cooker, ranging from entire pig joints with plenty of fat and connective tissue to leaner diced pork, pork mince, or loin. Each cut takes slightly different preparation or cooking times,.

How To Cook Beef

With deliberate effort and clean cooking , beef can make meals more tasteful and nutritious.

Lean beef is a naturally high source of several key vitamins and minerals. A three-ounce cooked portion of lean beef contains ten critical components, including protein, zinc, iron, and B vitamins.

Check out the advice and food safety suggestions below to help you incorporate beef into your healthy eating plan.

Beef is lean. A piece of cooked fresh meat is termed "lean" if it contains less than 10 grams of total fat, 4.5 grams of saturated fat, or 95 milligrams of cholesterol per 100 grams (3.5 ounces). Look for the words "round" or "loin" in the name to easily identify lean beef cuts. Some examples are sirloin, tenderloin, top loin, eye round, top round, round tip, bottom round, and flank. These can be sliced into roasts or steaks. The most common type of ground beef is 93 percent lean.

Trim away any visible fat from the cooked beef before serving Portion sizes. Beef is an excellent supplement to a balanced diet when eaten in moderation and in a lean cut.

Begin with a 3-ounce serving of lean beef (about the size of a deck of cards) and supplement with colorful vegetables, fruits, and nutritious grains.

Shopping for meat. When shopping for beef, remember to follow food safety guidelines. Remember to verify the "sell by" date to ensure it hasn't passed before purchasing. Moreso, before checking out, get some beef. Use separate plastic bags for raw beef to prevent cross-contamination with ready-to-eat meals if raw meat juice leaks. If it would take more than 30 minutes to receive your Purchased beef and store it in a cooler.

After purchase, refrigerate or freeze beef as soon as possible. A refrigerator set to 40°F or lower will keep most goods safe, but not permanently. Cool temperatures decrease bacterial development, but they do not completely stop it. Food should be consumed as soon as possible to maintain its quality and freshness. Raw hamburgers and other ground meats can be kept in the refrigerator for 1-2 days, raw roasts, steaks, and chops for 3-5 days, and cooked meat for 3-4 days. Remember to lay beef packages on the lowest level of the refrigerator, on a plate or tray, to catch fluids. Before freezing beef, label each packet with the date.

Name of cut, weight, or number of servings. This will surely enable you keep to the "first in, first out" rule.

To retain quality, follow these freezer storage guidelines:

3-4 months for raw hamburgers
and other ground meats.

 4-12 months for raw steaks and
roasts, and

 2-3 months for cooked meat.
Use a food thermometer to
ensure that food is cooked to a
safe minimum internal
temperature that will kill
hazardous microorganisms.
Steaks and roasts should be
cooked to 145°F and rested for 3
minutes. Allow the meat to rest
for the time provided once it has
been removed from the heat
source. During repose, the
temperature remains steady or
rises, destroying hazardous
germs.
Hamburgers produced from
ground beef should achieve
160°F and do not require rest
time.Be sure you freeze the

remaining portions between two to three hours of cookery.

CHAPTER 10
Apps and sweet

Easy crockpot appetizers that everyone will like. These mere delicious and nutritious formula will make it convenient to host your next party. These recipes for dips, meatballs, chicken wings, and more are delicious. There are so many excellent appetizer options. These slow-cooker appetizers are quick to prepare and require no effort. The hardest part is picking which appetizer recipe to try first.

They are ideal for sporting events, holidays, and celebrations. Each slow cooker recipe is incredibly simple and tasty.

Whether you're preparing for the big game or having a movie night at home, these appetizer ideas will be fantastic.

When learning how to create appetizers, you need first to understand what an appetizer is. Appetizer meals might include crisp salads and transparent soup recipes.

Seafood cocktails, fruit cups, or light canapés. These "teasers" are offered at the table before supper to stimulate the appetite. These are meticulously arranged in conjunction with the supper and serve as a foreshadowing of the next dinner.

Before dinner, appetizer recipes are always light, slightly more complicated, and served in individual portions. It is important to keep a few favorite easy appetizers on hand to cook when you are busy.

If a cocktail hour is scheduled before dinner, plates of appetizers can be passed around to be consumed with the drinks. These appetizer recipes must be finger foods that are easy to eat while standing. When arranging the appetizers, keep the cocktail hour in mind as well as the sort of dinner. If you're going to have a big supper, limit your appetizers. Don't overwhelm your guests with hefty appetizers before sitting down to dinner. Learn how to make appetizers for each meeting.

Avoid imagining your slow cooker is just for spicy meals. As these recipes show, a slow cooker can be your best friend for making a variety of sweets, from poached fruit to self-saucing puddings.

Why Should You Use a Slow Cooker for Desserts?

Many desserts benefit from extended, slow cooking to allow the flavors to combine and merge. Consider poached fruit, compotes, and creamy rice pudding. These are some tips that will make you a winner:

If you use poaching syrup for fruit like pears, quinces, or apples, don't discard the liquid once it's finished. It can be kept in the fridge for up to two weeks and can be used to poach another batch of fruit.

If you're making a sponge or pudding, don't open the lid during the cooking process since condensation will run down the sides of the cooker and leave moist spots on the top of the pudding.

To assist a steamed pudding to rise as it cooks, cover the steamer with a pleated paper lid followed by foil.

Vanilla beans are a common ingredient in slow-cooker sweets and can be reused for future dishes. Simply wash, dry thoroughly, and store.

Rice based pudding:

Allowing this dessert to slowly cook throughout the day eliminates the difficulty of producing the ideal rice pudding. Rice pudding, a popular dessert among both young and elderly, is great warm or cold and pairs well

with canned, fresh, or stewed
fruits. Alternatively, sprinkle a
little cinnamon and pour with
cream over the pudding.
Butterscotch Self-Saucing
Pudding
Creamed rice pudding is a
traditional slow cooker recipe.

Lemony pudding:

This cold-weather favorite is
simple to prepare in the slow
cooker, allowing you to plan
dessert well ahead of dinnertime.
Made straight into the slow
cooker dish, this dessert requires
no extra equipment and is easy to
clean up after.

Allow the custard to thicken up
for five minutes outside of the
cooker before serving.

chocolate pudding

A chocolate pudding is one of
the most popular winter desserts,
and it's even easier to make

ahead of time. Remember that the goal of a beautiful chocolate pudding is to strike an appealing balance between cake and custard, so cook these recipes until the top is just firm. Sprinkle icing sugar on top of the pudding and serve hot or warm with cream or ice cream.

Slow Cooker Chocolate Self-Saucing Pudding.

Slow Cooker Black Cherry and Chocolate Pudding

Moist Mud Pudding.

Custard desserts: Although we frequently believe that dairy and slow cookers do not mix, this recipe defies the odds and yield a creamy custard ideal for serving with canned, fresh, or stewed fruit. Slow-cooker baked custard.

OTHER RECIPES TO TRY

There are many different slow cooker sweets to attempt, so here are a few to get you started. If you want to experiment with your recipes, search for ones that benefit from lengthy, slow cooking, such as baked apples, bread puddings, or steamed puddings.